The Living Mala

By Nancy Alder
and

D1502121

This book is dedicated to everyone living their yoga.

Looking back, I have always "done" yoga. Not because my parents did it or because I grew up doing down-dogs or handstands. It is the "other" parts of yoga that I really remember doing. What I call pranayama now, in high school I called it my eight count breath to get sleep. What we call asana or poses in yoga, we just called our warm up exercises in massage therapy school. These simple tools that I have carried with me, like taking a pause for internal reflection before making a decision, are all parts of living a yoga practice. Over the years, I have been able to easily look back and say I have been practicing yoga long before I ever did a sun salutation.

When I became a mother for the first time, I was obsessed with learning how to do a handstand. I NEEDED to learn how to stand on my hands not because I wanted to teach my son, but more I wanted to do them with him. First of all, he was a baby when I had this obsession, so theoretically I had years before I really had to worry about it. Secondly, having just had a baby, handstands were off the table for awhile, period. So I turned inward. I started to use the time I was nursing my baby to meditate, to breathe, to be. I started again, to live the practice. Having children (I now have two boys), took me from vinyasa flows, saluting the sun, and arm balancing tries to stillness, turning inwards, feeling my breath. It brought me back to what yogis have really been searching for: to live a present life. ~ liz

My yoga mat created a way to carve out some space just for me. I began really practicing when my kids were very young; the ability to be alone and just breathe quietly was such a gift. I learned how to come back to being "Nancy" and not just "Mom." I remembered how to breathe when things were difficult and how to stretch when space became crowded. I was reminded that I have tools within myself to handle the challenges and joys that arise on a daily basis.

Later as my physical practice grew, I gained this fundamental awareness of my own strength –physical, spiritual and mental. Yoga helped me appreciate my body after two children and growing older. I understood that the practice was not merely in my arms and abdomen, legs and back. But that the inner work and fortitude I gained from the eight limbs of the practice were as important, or perhaps more so than all the arm balances I conquered. Today, my yoga changes with each moment. It shows up in my inhales and exhales, in my understanding of my inner dialog, in my relationships and in stillness. I move when my mind is too loud and sit when I need the space. My yoga is now all moments in my life. ~ nancy

What is a mala and why 108 beads?

A mala is a necklace used for meditation or ritual in many different practices. It is a strand of beads containing 108 beads and one additional bead, totem or icon considered the "guru bead." This special bead is in place not only to help those using the mala for counting, but also as a reminder of the teachers who have guided us on our path. Often the circle of the mala is closed merely at the guru bead. However, it may also contain a tassel for decoration at the end.

The practice of meditation using a mala is frequently one of repeating a phrase or mantra 108 times, with the individual moving along the length of the mala as they chant. Each bead represents a repetition of the chant and the mala serves as a reminder of their position in the counting of the chant. Upon reaching the guru bead, the meditator knows they have done 108 rounds of meditation, and then turns the mala clockwise while holding the guru bead or tassel and continues to the next round. It is customary to NOT pass the guru bead in the counting as a sign of respect for our teachers, and that is why the meditator rotates the mala between each 108 chants.

108 is a number used for mala bead necklaces for many reasons. You can choose which resonates most deeply with you, but here are just a few of the reasons why malas have 108 beads:

- In Sanskrit there are 54 letters, which each have a male and female version equaling 108 letters in total. It is noteworthy that many mantras are in or have their origins in Sanskrit.

- There are 108 energy lines within the body leading to the heart chakra or energy center.

- There are 108 sacred sites in India.

- The average distance from the moon or the sun to the Earth is 108 times their respective diameters.

Grab a seat, stand tall, or rest as you begin The Living Mala.

How does this book work?

This book is composed of 108 "beads" for creating a living practice with an extra "guru bead" to complete the circle of the mala. Start with the guru bead blessing each time as a way to honor yourself as teacher. These practices can be read from beginning at the first bead and moving one bead a day. Alternatively, read until a bead sparks something in you, or open to any page and trust you will get the bead that you need in that moment. No matter how you choose to use this book, we hope it will provide tools to continue to ignite your yoga as a life practice rather than just one on the mat. We hope that each time you choose one of these practices, you will glean something new. As you change so does your perception of these practices. You will be coming to each action from a different place, even if you have done it dozens of times in the past.

Just have fun and see if you can find within these pages a fresh viewpoint about your yoga practice and therefore, your life. These beads of practice are designed as a way to highlight how many of your already existing routines are indeed yogic in nature. It is our hope that you can also find a few new practices to add into everyday life from those that we have offered.

Guru Bead.

May I find peace in every day.
May I be at ease in my own skin.
May I know the calmness in my
breath.
May I find the exquisite in the
simple.
May I feel joy within myself.
May I stand grounded and strong.
May I be kind to myself and
others.
May I find meaning in the moment.

1.

Take a deep breath.

Take five to 10 breaths or make it a minute or two of breathing. No matter how you begin, a deep breath can change the way your day goes. Notice how breath shifts your day.

2.

Feel connected to the Earth.

Stand with your feet hips' distance apart in the grass, dirt, or sand. Pick up one toe at a time until all your toes are raised, the ball and heel of your feet are deeply connected to the ground. Observe how grounding that stance feels. Return your toes to the ground but resist gripping.

3.

**Wash your face and look
at yourself.**

See your eyes, nose, and
mouth. Coming from a place
of non-judgment and not
explaining/story telling, can
you really see yourself? Be
present with yourself for a
few minutes and see the
amazingness that is YOU.

4.

Practice controlled breathing.

Inhale for a count of four, pause in the fullness at the top of your breath for a count of two, exhale for a count of four, pause in the emptiness at the bottom of your breath for a count of two. Do this breathing 10 times and notice how your attention shifts away from your mind and to your body.

5.

Make a morning beverage.

Turn this routine into a moving meditation. Be present. Fill the water. Scoop the tea or coffee or slice the lemon. Notice the smell, the texture of the tools, and let the beverage create itself. Then let the sipping of that beverage be a meditation too. Feel the cup in your hand. Observe the temperature, smell, and texture of the drink. Take a sip to enjoy.

6.

Let music be your medicine.

Pick a song that resonates deeply and listen to it instead of the news in your car. Notice how that shifts your mood in a way that talk radio does not.

7.

Set an intention.

Take a few moments every morning to set an intention for your day before you get going on your routine. Just as we do before we practice in a yoga class, setting an intention can keep the focus on what needs to get done or what we want to create. Allow that intention to travel with you through your day.

8.

Write ten things that bring you joy.

Be mindful of a tendency to only list impactful and big items/moments/ successes. Instead, look for the smaller ones. See the joy in the small moments.

9.

Use every day routines as your practice.

Brush your teeth to remind yourself to speak your truth and to clean out the untruths. Wash your body and notice how physically strong you are. Chant "I am strong" with every scrub of your skin. Rinse away any stagnant thoughts or negative thinking when you wash your hair. Take actions that seem like routines and make them sources of empowerment.

10.

Take a walk and experience it.

Surround yourself in the sounds of the journey: the clinking of shoes on the ground, the birds and wind, or the crunching of the stones under your feet. Become aware of being aware.

11.

Spend a few minutes plotting your day.

Set aside time to eat, walk away from your desk, or take some deep breaths outdoors. Be sure to schedule quiet time with some form of meditation. Allow these moments to be smaller, more manageable, such as five or ten minutes. Sneaking in these periods throughout the day will help create a sense of balance as well as help keep you present.

12.

Sit before starting.

Before racing off to go somewhere in your car, sit for two minutes with your eyes closed and draw your attention to your breath. Feel the expansion of your ribs in your inhale and contraction on your exhale. Notice the balance or lack thereof between inhales and exhales. Be totally present in your breathing. See how this presence changes your experience of racing into one of steadiness and calm.

13.

Move your body.

Whether it is folding forward while the coffee is brewing or just a few stretches because you plan on taking class later, add movement throughout the day. See how it keeps the body fluid and tension at bay. Try doing cat/cows as you sit at your work desk: inhale bring your chest forward (cow), exhale draw your chest in and round your back (cat). Five minutes every day is better than 90 minutes twice a week. You can make it happen.

14.

Turn off to tune in.

Turn off your cell phone, computer and/or television for 30 minutes every day during a time when you might otherwise be distracted by them. Use that time to rest, read a book, or practice poses or meditation.

15.

Get into color meditation.

Grab a coloring book or print a coloring page you like from the internet. Sit without distractions and create something beautiful. Carefully select colors and be mindful about coloring in the lines if that feels right. Observe how something as simple as creating a picture can be meditation.

16.
Make a glitter jar.

Grab a jar with a tightly sealing lid. Fill the jar mostly full with clear water. Add three to four tablespoons of glitter. Close the lid completely. Shake the jar and mix the glitter and the water. Set the jar on the table or counter and watch the glitter return to the bottom. Let this exercise be a mindfulness practice.

17.

Sit every day for five minutes.

Set a timer, close your eyes and meditate. Meditation does not require special skills or a quiet mind. All you need to do is turn inwards and check in with how you are feeling. Try to see what seated position feels most comfortable. Perhaps add in some movement such as a twist or stretch. Yoga can be both the five-minute practice or the hour practice. Give yourself permission to do what you can and not what you feel you should do.

18.

Be mindful with your words.

Are you speaking the truth?
Your truth? Being honest does
not mean being rude or hurtful.
Use your best judgment of what
you speak and do so with
thought of what you are saying
and how you are saying it.
Awareness is a simple way to
practice your yoga.

19.

Tune in.

Find a comfortable seat, close
your eyes, and place your
hands at your heart. What are
you longing for? What do you
really need right now to feel
whole? To feel connected? To
fill your cup? Listen for and to
the answers. They may not
come right away, which is ok.
Keep asking and listening.
Keep a journal nearby. When
the answers come to you, write
them down to remember.

20.

Practice walking meditation.

Start by connecting your feet to the ground on an exhale and stepping on an inhale. Walk as slowly as you breathe. Do not worry how far you go, simply go at the pace of your breath.

21.

Try seated sun breaths.

Sun breaths are a way to link your breath and movement from a seated position. Do 10 seated sun breaths: Raise your arms overhead on an inhale and bring your palms together and down the center of your body to your heart on your exhale. Inhale and fill up, exhale and release. Repeat at least 10 times.

22.

**Buy or pick flowers for
yourself or someone else.**

Notice how this simple gesture
changes the energy around
you.

23.

Take time to cool down with your breath.

If you are too hot, try this cooling breath work: Curl your tongue and breathe through your mouth. Inhale through your mouth, feeling the cool air on your tongue and exhale out your nose. A few rounds of this breath work will have you chill in no time. Unable to curl your tongue? Stick it out instead as you inhale. This mouth formation has the same benefits and cooling sensation*.

*Note: If you have low blood pressure, refrain from doing this breathing technique. Instead, practice long exhales.

24.

**Actively participate in the
creation of a salad.**

Mindfully cut each component into
similarly sized pieces, notice the
texture of the lettuce as you tear it
into smaller parts, consider the
quantity of cheese, meat and/or
dressing rather than merely
adding it without thought. Let the
making of a meal be a meditation.

25.

Take a stand.

Whether you are waiting in line at the grocery store, post office, or just getting up from your desk at work, rooting the feet down is a great yoga practice. With both feet on the floor, shift side to side between the right and left foot. Slow that movement down and find a spot that feels centered. Now shift your weight forward and backward. Slow down and return to center. Stay still. Close your eyes and take few breaths to tap into the sensation of standing.

26.

Create a sacred space for practice.

Fill it with things you love: flowers, photos of people who you love or are inspired by, Buddha/Mother Mary/Shiva or whoever represents your higher power. Add crystals, candles, or anything else you deem important to you. Make it large enough to unroll your mat or put your cushion down to meditate, and leave some room to move. Breathe in your sacred space.

27.

Do half sun salutations with chair pose.

Stand tall, inhale your arms overhead. Exhale, fold forward over bent knees and extend your arms behind you like a speed skater. Inhale up into chair pose. Exhale into a forward fold. Inhale your arms back up to standing. Exhale your hands to your heart. Repeat at least five times.

28.

Make a nature mandala.

Collect items from nature in your yard or at a park. Look for leaves, petals, stones, seeds, feathers. Use these treasures to create a mandala. A mandala is a circular design with both sides being mirror images of each other. Place petals, or stones of the same size/color in a pattern that looks special to you. Watch how things you sometimes overlook can create astonishing beauty.

29.

Heat up with Lion's Breath.

If staying warm is your challenge, try some lion's breath to get warm. Inhale through the nose, exhale out the mouth with your tongue sticking out and a releasing a "haaaaaa" sound. A few rounds of this energizing breathing technique and you are bound to feel warmer and stronger. Do not be afraid to really let out your roar*.

*Note: avoid on this practice if you have low blood pressure.

30.

Take in the sounds of morning.

Wake up and sit on your front step or porch. Listen for the sounds of the morning: birds, wind, traffic, children, rain, etc. Let this symphony of life be the music that provides a soundtrack for your day. Notice how these simple sounds have a complexity when they are combined.

31.

Find your seat.

Find a comfortable position that works for your body. Wiggle, shrug, and find what center feels like for you. Open and close your mouth to relax your jaw, bring your ears over your shoulders. Soften shoulders, firm the belly. Close your eyes and breathe. This seat is your comfortable one; remember that for class or at home.

32.

Slow down and be present.

There is a beauty in being present with one task at a time. Focusing on one thing at work or home offers you a chance to fully be present. Just as when we are moving through our practice on the mat, we need to give our full attention to one job. Use focus to increase your efficiency and accuracy.

33.

Meditate with a mudra.

Mudras are hand gestures which are a form of yoga. Bring your hands together in lotus mudra. Place your palms together and then gently create some space in the middle of the palms, except for the heel of the hands, while the pinky fingers and thumbs connect. Open the other fingers out widely like lotus petals. Set your hands at your heart chakra, or center of your chest. Take 10-20 breaths with your hands in this mudra inviting in truth and balance.

34.

Switch from routine to ritual.

Most days feel like routine rather than something extraordinary. This truth has more to do with how we see things rather than how things actually are. Take mundane acts and find the divine in them. Allow vacuuming to be a clearing. See dusting or wiping away dirt off the counters, as shifting the energy of your space. Look at laundry as starting fresh. What daily acts can be divine?

35.

Have a solo dance party.

Turn on some of your favorite dance songs. Play that music loudly in your living room or kitchen and dance. Dance in a way that makes you smile and brings you joy. Let the music move you.

36.

Find a place to sit for a few minutes.

Grab some headphones or earbuds to quiet outside noise. Close your eyes with your earbuds/headphones on and begin to listen to the music of your breath. Feel the texture of your breath and see how it changes the sound you are hearing. Practice turning inward with your attention as you quiet that noises outside of you.

37.

Wring out the stuck.

Like wringing out a washcloth, we can twist out the stuff that is stuck in our bodies. Think of twisting as a way to flush cells and our organs. Choose a gentle pose like reclined twist, which uses the movement of the lower body to twist. Allow gravity to do some work for you. Lying on the back, knees bent, drop the legs to the left side and open arms out into "T." Stay for a few breaths. On an exhale, return to your back and draw knees into chest before switching sides.

38.

Open a random book to any page.

Grab a book off your bookshelf and open up to a random page. Look at the first full sentence on that page. Write it down or read it out loud. How does it resonate with your life today? What words stick out for you? Observe how something seemingly unrelated to you can feel relevant and important.

39.

Cook/bake with intention.

Place the ingredients/tools on the counter in an easy to see fashion. Close your eyes for a moment and get focused. Inhale, exhale and open your eyes. Think about who you are nourishing with this meal. Think about the energy we receive from the foods we eat. Imagine filling this meal with love on every level: from dicing veggies to sautéing to boiling water. Feel gratitude for all the hands that helped get this food to you, farmers to grocery or market clerks. Thank yourself for taking the time to cook or bake. Enjoy the meal which is infused with love.

40.

**Take part in conscious
breath.**

Lie on your back and place a
yoga block or a medium weight
book on your abdomen.
Observe how the block/book
rises on your inhale and lowers
on your exhale. Try shifting the
pattern of your breath to one of
longer inhales or exhales or
alternatively, balanced inhales
and exhales. How does the
rhythm of the block change?
How do these differing
breathing patterns make you
feel?

41.

Do what you love.

We all have responsibilities. If your job is not exactly your dream job you do not have to stop doing what you love. Whether you have a secret dream to be a dancer or an artist or professional house flipper, start today to make that dream a reality. Little steps every day will help you feel some of that joy as you work toward what you love. If you already adore your job or are not really sure that you have found your path, start exploring new hobbies. Sign up for a sewing class, rocking climbing course, or simply go out and try something different. Having an activity you love doing every day will bring you more joy and presence in your life.

42.

Be still and observe.

Pour yourself a glass of seltzer.
Watch the bubbles rise until the
water is still.

43.

Flip your perspective.

You do not have to have an active inversion practice to change your point of view. Any shape that puts your heart over your head will do. Headstand, handstand, downward facing dog, supported bridge, or try putting your legs up the wall. Sit as close to the wall as possible and stretch your legs up the wall as you lie down near it. Changing your view can provide a shift in your day.*
*Make sure you listen to your body and acknowledge what you are able to do before doing it. Remember: do not do a hand or headstand if you have never done it with supervision from a teacher before, stick to something easier.

44.

Post one positive thing on social media a day for a week.

See if you can encourage friends to do the same. Create a virtual wave of positivity through your community.

45.

Listen for the bell to finish ringing.

Use a Tibetan singing bowl, Tingsha bells or use an online source to create the sounds of these instruments. Ring these instruments and observe how long the bells/ring goes until there is no sound. Repeat and listen for the end of the bell. Notice if you want to end this exercise when the faintest hint of bell is still ringing. Do not stop. Wait until the bell/bowl is completely done ringing. Notice the sound of no bell ringing

46.

Write your ideal day.

While yoga asks us to be as present as possible, it does not encourage living life blindly into the future. A helpful activity is to sit down and write how you want a day to look. Sit with pen to paper when you feel "off track" or need a reminder of what you are accomplishing. Plan out a work day and a free day from waking up to going to bed. What do these days look like? Is this in six months? A year? You can be as detailed as you want to be or just list out how the day will be spent as if it were already your calendar. Read through it and let it sink into your mind. It is where you want to be. This day is where you are heading.

47.

Make a happy playlist/

Take ten songs that make you smile no matter what is going on in your life. Share this playlist with friends or family. Play these songs in your car or home. Let music bring you joy.

48.

Take some time for some stillness.

Find a comfortable seat, use a cushion, a blanket, a block to sit on, or sit in a chair. Close your eyes and focus on your breathing. Slow your inhale down, let your exhale match. Take five of these intentional breaths. Inhale and picture the breath moving up the spine up to the crown of your head. Exhale out the mouth and imagine it also coming out of the third eye, between the eyebrows. Inhale again from the base of the spine to the crown of the head, exhale out the mouth and visualizing out of the third eye. Take three more of these spine and mind-rinsing breaths. Finally, inhale and exhale as normal. Open your eyes and take a moment to just breathe before moving.

49.

**Take some conscious
breaths.**

Bring your hands to the sides of
your torso near your lowest
ribs. Close your eyes and
observe how your ribs move
out and up on your inhale, in
and down on your exhale.
Continue with this breath
awareness by noticing the
texture and shape changes that
occur as you breathe. Contrast
and compare the way your
abdomen is soft and pliable and
your ribcage stiff and
structured. Observe how your
breath affects both locations.
Use breath awareness to be
present.

50.

Believe.

What do you believe in? God? Shiva? Allah? Mother Nature? Science? Take time to explore what you consider essential and try to incorporate time to trust in it every day. Connecting to what you believe is a great way to experience yoga and bring some spirituality to your day.

51.

Take in the sun.

On a sunny day, turn all the lights off in your house and allow only the brightness of the sun to light your space. See how the power of the sun can shift your energy. Watch how the light can bring warmth and happiness.

52.

Clean mindfully.

Brushing your teeth, washing
your face, drinking water, all
these things are ways to keep
clean. Sweating can be
cleansing. Meditation, eating
whole foods, laughing, and
crying all can be a practice of
cleaning. Take time each day to
feel clean, both energetically
and physically.

53.

Write a letter to yourself in six months.

Congratulate yourself on something you plan to achieve and on the success you have in doing that action. Make sure this success is a goal and something you plan to do. Be very detailed. Outline your successful steps to completing this achievement. Fill the letter with praise because you HAVE accomplished it successfully. Put the letter in an envelope and tape it to the calendar six months from today, or set a reminder on your phone, when you will open it. Allow yourself to be congratulated about your success.

54.

Choose Meditation.

You can find five minutes to mediate. To meditate, you do not have to be sitting. Meditation can be making mindful steps from one room to the next, present in mind and body. It can be gazing out the window at nature, being present and aware. It can be an eyes-closed dance party, feeling your body move through space and taking in the rhythm of the music. Meditation as a seated practice is great, but do not feel bound by that style. Bring awareness, presence, and a clear mind to any action and BOOM: you are meditating.

55.

Create some spa water.

Combine fresh purified water with cucumbers, mint, basil, or citrus. Place this spa water in a clean, clear glass. Drink the whole glass with the intention that you are treating yourself to a spa moment. Let yourself enjoy the luxury of this healthy water and the joy of spoiling yourself. Create a container of your favorite flavor to keep in the refrigerator for moments you need a treat.

56.

Practice shoulder shrugs.

Sit in a comfortable position. Inhale, spread the space in your upper back. Draw your shoulders together and up towards your ears. Exhale, draw your shoulders down the back. Next inhale and spread the space across the lower half of your upper back. Draw your armpits towards each other in the back of the body and exhale drawing them down your back. Finally inhale and expand the space across the lowest part of your middle back. Bring your elbows to your sides and forearms/hands out to the side away from your body. Draw the bottom tips of the shoulder blades together and slowly guide them down your back on an exhale. Repeat three times. Observe the tension dissolve in your shoulders and back.

57.

Do a driving meditation.

When you are driving in traffic and are fully stopped at a light or when you arrive at your destination, try a short meditation. Take a moment. Inhale fully, exhale out the mouth. Inhale fully, exhale and say to yourself: "I am content." Inhale fully, exhale and say to yourself: "I am connected." Inhale fully, exhale and say to yourself: "I am love." Inhale fully, exhale slowly.

58.

Be mindful with your food.

If we are what we eat, what are
you putting into your body?
Food is fuel as well as
pleasure, so take a good hard
look at what you are eating.
What do you like? Do you
reward yourself a lot with treats
or snacks between meals? Are
you drinking enough water?
Bringing awareness to our plate
is a great way to help you
notice if you feel sluggish after
a meal or if you're snacking
when in reality you are just
thirsty. Notice your habits when
it comes to meals and food.

59.

Put your feet up.

After a long day, there is nothing like shifting energy by raising your feet. Putting our feet up tells our body it is time to move into relaxation mode. Legs up the wall takes that idea a step further, because it allows for the reverse movement of energy and blood flow. This practice draws down your energy towards your heart and allows your circulatory system to rest. Legs up the wall is the basic of all inversions and is a great way to end the day.

60.

Practice breath awareness.

Breathe in and know that you are breathing in. Breath out and know that you are breathing out.

61.

Make an essential oil mist.

Combine 10 drops of your
favorite essential oil or
combination of oils with distilled
water in a small spray bottle.
Spray to clear the energy of
your space or above your head
to carry the scent with you all
day.

62.

Be a good listener.

Our days are filled with conversations. Some of these chats are important and many that are not. Nevertheless, our presence is being requested by another person. Instead of allowing your mind to drift off into your to-do list or what you want to say when it is your turn, really listen to what is being said. Take in their physical cues, what their body is telling you. Hear their words and hold space for what is being said. Then, speak from the heart when the time arrives. Being a good friend, partner, or employee/employer starts with being present and really listening.

63.

Buy a stranger a coffee.

Pay for the person behind you
in line or in the car after you.
Feel how that good gesture
changes your day and imagine
how it affects them positively
too.

64.

Give thanks.

Say "please," say "thank you."
Offer a "you are welcome." If
you never say another mantra
or prayer, these three phrases
will be enough. Ask kindly, give
gratitude for what you receive,
or offer joy in giving.

65.

Practice a meditation with mudra.

Take both hands and begin pressing fingers to your thumbs like this: First finger and thumb come together on both hands. Then middle finger to thumb, ring finger to thumb and pinky to thumb. First get a sense of the rhythm of this action. Then draw your attention to the temperature, pressure and texture as you meet fingers and thumbs and as you separate them. Do five to 10 rounds of this mudra meditation.

66.

Meet the sun or greet the moon.

We are not all morning people, but there is something magical and beautiful about watching the sunrise. Likewise, the sunset is something we cherish whether we spend those last few moments of the day. So chose one, sunrise or sunset, and watch it every day for a week. Notice how calm that practice can be, whether you are greeting the day or saying "goodnight." Enjoy the beauty only nature can provide.

67.

Leave space for bliss.

You have practiced how to set
time aside in your schedule, so
make some of that time for
bliss. Maybe you want to enjoy
a special piece of chocolate
after a particularly not-fun
meeting, or a walk to your
favorite place to watch the
birds, bliss can be found in the
small moments. Slow down to
appreciate them.

68.

Let it go.

We cannot do everything in one day. There are only 24 hours to be had. We need to sleep, to eat food, to do our work. So what in your schedule can you release? What part of your day can you simplify? How can you make your day smoother? How can the transitions be more mindful? Drop what is not working and embrace your day.

69.

Take a photo of yourself smiling.

Without a moment's thought, share it on social media. Try not to judge or critique yourself. Be happy in the confidence that you are you.

70.

Mindfully make avocado toast.

Grab your favorite bread and place it in the toaster or toaster oven until it reaches desired crispness. Slice up a ripe avocado and place that on the toasted bread. Add spices, sauces, seeds, or greens of your choice. Choose to add brightness such as lime juice or spiciness such as hot pepper flakes. Enjoy the combination of decadence and healthiness.

71.

Wait to look at your phone.

Being able to look at your phone first thing is an amazing way to connect to the world. Technology is incredible and useful. Today, do not give up your technology, but instead try connecting to yourself first. Take time to be an active participant in your morning instead of seeing what you missed from last night. Simply enjoy your routine and connecting to you. Later over coffee or after breakfast, check to see what the world is up to; it will still be there waiting for you.

72.

Create a self massage ritual.

Take a bottle of water and pour a small amount out into a favorite plant. Then place the partially full bottle in the freezer until it is completely frozen (12-24 hrs). Use the frozen water bottle as a massage tool on hot days for your upper back or feet. Gently roll the frozen water bottle in places where tightness and tension linger.

73.

Inhale and Ahhhhh.

Take a deep breath in, exhale loudly. Do it again, inhale and exhale loudly. Add some length to the exhale and see how that shifts things. Now inhale and exhale loudly while shaking your body. What does movement add to your breathing?

74.

Become aware of all your senses.

Grab a pencil or pen. Write down one favorite thing for each sense. For example: smell: oranges; taste: spicy. Imagine that you are experiencing each of those things in that moment. Notice how this awareness offers you a chance to become present in your body and allow your mind to quiet.

75.

Fold Forward.

Even if you are not trying to become more flexible, touching your toes is good for you. Cannot touch your toes? Try bringing your hands into the crooks of your elbows, then fold and release. Make sure you keep a slight bend in your knees as you fold to keep your low back safe. Try this position first thing in the morning or right before bed. Fold forward and stay there for five breaths. Inhale, bend knees and come all the way up to standing with a flat back.

76.

Take in the sounds of your day.

We often feel uncomfortable in silence, but truly it is a rarity for our world to be totally quiet. From birds chirping as the morning breaks to the sound of wind or cars in the middle of the night, there is almost always a little hum in our days. Even the computers we use make noises if you listen. Take a pause through out your day to close your eyes and really hear. You'll be surprised at how nice the "quiet" can be when you experience it.

77.

Notice your strength and connections.

Sit in a comfortable position and close your eyes. Turn your awareness to the outer edges of your body. Feel how your container is separate from the air and space around you. Imagine that you have a thick black marker in your hand. Draw an imaginary line around the outer shape of your body. Now bring your attention back to the separateness of your container and the space/people/things around you. Finally, retrace your steps backward and imagine that you are erasing that thick black imaginary line around yourself. Feel how you are still strong and intact in your container, but are also able to connect with the outside world at the same time.

78.

Make an indoor garden.

Grab some succulents, some
herbs, or some flowers. Take
an old bowl, or even a jar, to
turn into a planter. Let your
fingers get dirty, taking time to
tend to the roots of your new
friends. Mindfully care for this
living being every day, talking
to it, and remembering that we
all need a little water, sunshine,
and good roots to grow.

79.

Trust in yourself.

Trust that you are important.
Trust that you are worthy.
Trust that you belong.

80.

Give a big OK.

Start using the Gyan or OK mudra when you agree with friends. The Gyan mudra looks a lot like saying OK with our hands, pointer finger to the thumb with the other three fingers extended. When you are responding to a friend and using this mudra, you are confirming with life that all is good, peaceful, and calm. Create that sensation of goodness, peacefulness, and calmness with your hands.

81.

Spend time with a pet you love.

See how animals are so present when they are with you and cultivate that presence with them. Take that experience with you when you are with people. Be present with all beings.

82.

Create space for the things you love.

Each room of your home should have bits and pieces that remind you of great trips, friends and family you love, and treasures you have come across on your path. Create little altars, or just a place to set these things so that your eyes will find them when you look around the room. Bringing a smile to your day by remembering these special moments through these tokens.

83.

Do a seated twist.

Sit cross-legged and place your hands on heart. Close your eyes and feel the movement of your breath under your hands. Inhale and lengthen your spine. Exhale and twist your torso to the right. Keep your hands on your heart. Inhale back to center. Exhale and twist your torso to the left. Inhale back to center. Continue with this moving and breathing twist for five more times to each side.

84.

Create a rain cup.

When rain is on the horizon, set a glass or a bowl out to catch it. Place it someplace that you can watch as the water fills and take a moment to give thanks for this awesome element, then use it to water a indoor plant in need of some water or pour it back to the earth.

85.

Say hello everyone.

A simple smile, nod, or hello to
those you see throughout your
day can not only brighten up
someone else's day, it can also
help you feel seen and heard
too. Getting into the practice of
saying hello and seeing your
surroundings and community
will help you feel more
connected to those around you.

86.

Experience the bounty of a harvest.

Go to your local farmer's market or out to your own garden and find fresh, ripe foods to enjoy. Sit down and close your eyes. Take a bite and notice the smell/taste/texture. Let the juice run down your chin and enjoy the simplicity of a ripe fruit or vegetable.

87.

Practice dry brushing.

Use a stiff bristle brush. Before bathing, brush your dry skin working always back towards the heart. From wrist to shoulder, ankle to hip. Be mindful of areas with lymph nodes. Brush all points on the legs and arms, back and belly. Make this lymphatic stimulation practice a daily ritual.

88.

Create a collection.

Grab a clean mason jar. Fill it
with a collection of natural
things you have gathered in a
favorite place: sea glass, ocean
rocks, feathers. Place it in your
home somewhere you look
often to remind you of moments
you love.

89.

Be present with pleasures.

Enjoy a piece of dark chocolate. Rather than eat it quickly, savor the experience. Be mindful of how you open the package. Notice the texture of the wrapping. Feel the hardness of the chocolate and the smoothness or bumpiness of its surface. Place the chocolate in your mouth and observe the sensations that come with flavor. Allow the chocolate to dissolve over time and not by chewing. Let the flavor linger as it melts and truly experience the bliss.

90.

Try practicing yoga a new way.

Lie on your belly. A reverse corpse pose is a great way to soften as well as explore having the pressure of the earth on your front body. Notice where your body touches the ground and where it arches. Slow your breath and enjoy doing this different perspective on relaxation.

91.

Create your own warmth.

Rub your hands together,
creating heat in your hands.
When you feel the warmth,
place your hands on your face.
Hold them there until the heat
dissolves. Rub your hands
together again, building energy.
This time place them some
place that needs some love:
your heart, back, knees, or
somewhere else you wish to
send warmth.

92.

Allow creativity to inspire you.

Add some doodling into your day. You do not have to be an artist to let pen and paper create something. Take a deep breath, clear your mind and let the drawing instrument swirl or create shapes. Doodling is a great exercise in letting go of expectations. Allow yourself to be surprised by what you create.

93.

Practice constructive rest.

Lie on your back with your knees bent and feet on the floor. Place your feet at least a foot from the base of your spine. Close your eyes. Draw your attention to the lower back and feel the space between your back and the floor. Stay in this position, called "constructive rest" for 10-20 minutes. At the end of the 10-20 minutes return your attention to your lower back. Be aware how the arch of this area is less.
Notice gravity and relaxation have filled the space in your back.

94.

Care for your crystals.

Gather your favorite crystals and place them in a bowl. On full moon and new moon nights set the bowl of crystals in a window sill or outside for charging (new moon) or cleansing (full moon). Imagine that you are filling them with manifestation energy with the new moon and you are releasing from the crystals anything you no longer need on the full moon.

95.

Watch the weather.

If it is rainy, snowy, windy, or a
perfect day, take a moment to
just soak in what is happening
around you. Appreciate the
freshness that weather offers.

96.

Practice Abhaya mudra.

Sit in a comfortable position. Raise your right arm and bend at your elbow with your palm facing outward. This mudra is called "Abhaya mudra" and represents fearlessness. With your hand in Abhaya mudra breathe in steadiness and breathe out struggle. Breathe in bravery, breathe out fear. Breathe in knowing, breathe out uncertainty.

97.

Let it go.

Write down at least five things you are ready to release. This list can be items or actions you wish to no longer have/do. Then tear this list into as many small pieces as possible, removing these things from your presence with each tear. Feel the lightness that has come from letting them go.

98.

Wear something you love.

Choose a color you find
soothing or energizing and
where it on a day you need a
little pick me up. Notice how it
feels to draw that color into
your day. See how choice can
invite in soothing or energizing
qualities.

99.

Make a gratitude jar.

Pick a favorite vase and place it by your bedside. Put a pad of paper and some pens there as well. Tear a small piece of paper off the pad and write down something you were grateful for that day. Place that paper in the vase. Commit to doing this exercise every night for a month. On the first day of the next month read what you were grateful for and remember.

100.

Take the yoga pose: bound angle.

Bring the soles of your feet together: heel to heel, ball of foot to ball of foot. Place pillows under the knees if you need some support. Feeling the sitting bones and balancing pressure on each side. Bring the palms of the hands together in prayer at the heart, pushing evenly from one hand into the other. Notice the sensations that are happening as you connect your hands and feet. Slow your breath, close your eyes and feel.

101.

Make and release tension.

Interlace your hands with palms together. Squeeze your hands together as tightly as you possibly can. Invite in all the tension you have including the fears, anxiety and anger. Imagine you are squeezing them between your palms. Now take a long exhale and release the fingers and place your hands palm to palm, fingers touching but not intertwined, letting fear and anxiety go. Observe the ease and freedom you feel. Take ten breaths with your hands in this position.

102.

Have a laugh out loud moment.

Laughing is a great way to clear energy and can be a beautiful gift of bliss. Whether watching a short video of puppies playing or listening to your favorite comedian, or participating in a good old fashioned tickle war, laughing is a great way to feel content and clear energy.

103.

**Let something green show
you life.**

Place a small plant in a window
where you look out frequently.
See it as a reminder to live
fully.

104.

Have a sing-a-long.

Play your favorite song, sing a-long and let the music move you. Find a song with lyrics that inspire you. Let the words and the music move you. Imagine that you are the singer. Watch how music and words are powerful agents of energy.

105.

Stand in Mountain Pose.

Place your feet hip distance apart. Stand with your hands by your sides, arms slightly outstretched, and fingers spread. Feel connected to the earth. Feel strong and steady. Feel like a mountain.

106.

Relax your tight areas.

Soften your jaw. Soften your shoulders. Unclench your teeth.

107.

Make sun tea.

Find a large clear jar or pitcher with a lid. Fill it nearly full with purified, cold water. Select 3-5 tea bags of your favorite tea blend. Place the tea bags in the jar and close the lid. Leave the pitcher outside in the sun. Watch as the heat of the sun transforms two things (water and tea) into one: sun tea.

108.

Write some self love notes.

Leave love notes to yourself. Little reminders of your wit or kindness are easy ways to be aware of who you are and what you love about yourself. Be reminded that we all have many great attributes. Leaving little love notes to yourself is a way to tell yourself about those qualities.

These 108 practices are a gateway to exploring how yoga can be not only a daily practice, but available in small, incremental doses. We hope you have seen that yoga is not defined by a mat, a studio or poses. But rather, your yoga can come in the form of being fully present during any moment during your day. You can practice your yoga when you breathe, you think before reacting, you appreciate and when you communicate. Your yoga practice therefore is not limited to merely a pose or these 108 actions, but anything throughout your day when you are aware and present. This book is a reminder that you are indeed living your yoga, and is merely a jumping off point for acknowledging that truth.

~NOTES~

~NOTES~

~NOTES~

~NOTES~

~NOTES~

~NOTES~

~NOTES~

~NOTES~

~NOTES~

For more information about The Living
Mala, please contact Nancy and
Eliazbeth at eightlimblife@gmail.com or
at http://eightlimblife.com

Nancy Alder: www.flyingyogini.com

Elizabeth Vartanian:
www.blissfulbetty.com

Acknowledgements:

We would both like to thank our yoga students for being our teachers, for trusting us, for showing up and allowing us to hold their space. Thank you to the eight limb life community and students who have been a continual source of inspiration and for living your yoga. Thank you to Christina Nicole and Elizabeth Rowan for giving our first online course a look and feedback. We are grateful to Anna Guest-Jelly for an early edit of this book and for her wise and helpful suggestions. Without you all, we would still be editing and editing and editing! ~NA EV

~~

First and foremost, I have to thank my partner and co-author, Nancy. Woman you inspire me, you challenge me, and without you, this book would be just an article on my laptop. To say that you are the cream to my coffee is an understatement, thank you for balancing out all my "crazy" ideas. Thank you for all the phone calls, text messages, and emails to support not only this book, but also my motherhood dramas and the growth of myself as a yogi and human.

To my community of yoga peeps here in Austin, this book is for you! Thank you for showing up to your practice and to yourself every week. To my Once Over community, thank you for being my "first students" in the tree house, thank you for the amazing coffee and the great conversations.

To my teachers who are far too many to name, but a special thank you to Erinn Lewis and Mark Heron for the continual open arms, encouragement, and the support in all I teach. Thank you to Kara Pendl and Mel Frontino, you BOTH showed up at the right time and helped me bloom. I can never thank you enough. To Liz Davis, thank you for being my writing partner. Our hours of talking, sharing, and sipping coffee have been priceless to me. To all the yogis around the globe that I have connected with through social media, huge huge hugs to you! A special shout out to: Christina I adore you, Elizabeth Rowan you are an alchemist, Lo my international yoga mystery woman. May our connections continue and our work to share the love be strong.

To my parents, I love you and thank you for always encouraging me to grow and challenge myself. Thank you for raising me to be independent and strong. To my siblings, guys I love you. Thanks for encouraging, teasing, hanging out and enjoying beers together. Family, I love you!!

To my lady tribe: Rhokel Normington, Robin Chambers, and Karla DeLong, thank you! You are always in my heart and you will always be. To Bug and Bear, you both are my teachers, my heart and soul. I love you both to the moon and back. This book and so much of my yoga or writing is inspired by you both, you two will always be my teachers and my loves. And because you picked last, to my partner Matt, you are my rock and without your constant love, encouragement, jokes, and support along with your amazing proof reading skills! I would be no where without you, thank you so much. Babe you made this happen ~Elizabeth Vartanian

~~

I am eternally grateful to Liz for being not only my co-creator for eight limb life, but my co-author and chief cheerleader on this book. Her ability to work hand in hand with me, and to push me in her gentle but supportive way to make it happen has been invaluable. Being able to talk to her via text or phone every day during this process and for many years has been a giant gift. She is my sister from another mister and I couldn't ask for a better partner and friend.

I want to thank my mentor and friend Dani Shapiro for reminding me that I can do this crazy thing called "writing" and giving me tools to make it happen. I am grateful for all the women who gave me constructive feedback on my writing during Dani's retreats and for their creative inspiration. Your words are nourishment, truly.

In no particular order I am grateful for these folks because:

Anna Guest-Jelly shows me that sharing what moves you and smiling big are exaaaaactly what the doctor ordered.

Sharon Cormier was there first with such grace and humility that she opened the door to even envisioning this book. Diane Quinn keeps me writing and coffee filled. Christine Jablonski always gives me the straight story and totally understands my love of great wine and wise teachers and will happily commiserate with me during every hot, humid day. Michelle Martello reminds me that being smart, business savvy and fun are attainable and won't break the bank. Kate Bartollota has been a great source of help in the details and shows me a woman is a force to be reckoned with no matter what obstacles present themselves. Jennifer Draeger is my first cyber soul-sister and was the reason I started this whole writing and social media journey which lead me to meet Liz. Jennilyn Carson of YogaDork opened her internet pages to my words, and thereby many doors for me. Jen Heseltine and Elle Podgorsky Courtney are my fellow bad eggs who make me laugh, show me strength and understand what I'm thinking even if I just give them a glance. Stacy and Seth Newfeld for understanding family does not need to include shared genes.

Heather and Marc Titus, Sarah Russell and Nikki Levine gave me the first opportunities to teach eight limb life ideas to yoga students in person. Justine Fuller, Mindy Porrell, Jessica Tracy, Anne Crone, Laura Crane, Shelly Bigda and Cherie Trice trusted me to teach their students safely and often. Maranda Pleasant gave me the opportunity to get my words in print for the first time and to help those dear to me do so also.

My yoga teachers Anne Falkowski, Jude Kochman, Matt Falkowski, Joe Barnett, Jillian Pransky, Cheri Clampett, Arturo Peal, Sadie Nardini, Rolf Gates and Heidi Sormaz inspired me, taught me and lit so many fires. My students are safe, supported and love yoga because of you.

My social media tribe of yogis, writers, moms, dads, women and men who have reached out, shared, liked and commented on my posts for over eight years. You have allowed me into your worlds and reminded me that what I have to say is important. I am eternally grateful for your continued support and connections. You have lifted me up in so many ways. I hope to give you all a hug in person one day.

I want to thank my family. My parents Carl and Jeannette who not only talk me off the ledge deftly when I need it, but are always there to support me, encourage me and help me in any way. My brother Steve reminds me to get my vaccinations, to laugh and is one of the greatest guys ever. He never gives up and that motivates me too. My mother-in-law Joan for her kindness, patience and raising a stellar man whom I was able to marry. My late father-in-law Mark for his giant heart, his generosity, and his ability to commiserate with me when everyone else was late but we were on time.

The furry elf keeps us all laughing, loved and in line. I'm grateful she doesn't mind being a stand in for the human elves and getting her picture taken.

I am so overwhelmed with love and gratitude for my elves who have put up with me sharing their stories but not their names for so many years. They remind me every single day that laughter, love and lots of deep breaths are the medicine I need most. Without them I am not sure I would be a yoga teacher or a writer. They are my gurus.

Finally, there is not enough space in any book or acknowledgment to thank my guy Nathan. Through 20 years he has stuck by my side, dealing with my craziness and unusual professions. He has supported me by making anything I want to do possible and by being the best father to the elves. He has cooked glorious meals, listened to me rant and rave and still manages to smile. Mostly he has loved me no matter what and has kept me laughing every single day of those 20 years. This book is for him. ~Nancy Alder

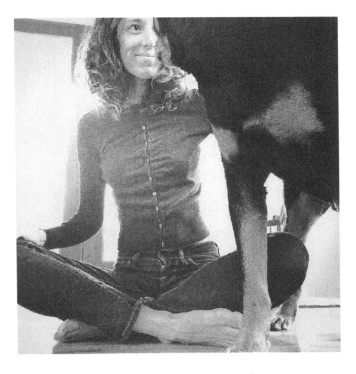

Elizabeth Vartanian is a yoga teacher,
writer and mama in Austin, TX. Her
carefully crafted classes include a loving
blend of restorative and yin yoga,
myofascial release, along with space to
come "home" to your body. The soft
surrender of restorative offer yogis a
chance to leave class feeling energized
and supported. Liz's classes feel like a
community and students are often

surprised with home cooked goodies after long relaxing savasanas. Her training with viniyoga teachers during her 200-hr has offered her a chance to lead yoga practices with authenticity and heart but, from a place of safety and knowledge. Liz's playful attitude keeps her class fun, challenging, and always full of laughter! Liz is a writer whose work was recently featured in OM Yoga Magazine. The delicate balance she strikes as a yoga teacher and mom was highlighted in Origin Magazine. She is an avid stand up paddle boarder and Instagram video maker. When not teaching yoga, Liz can be found with her family where there is coffee, good friends, toy trucks and a body of water!

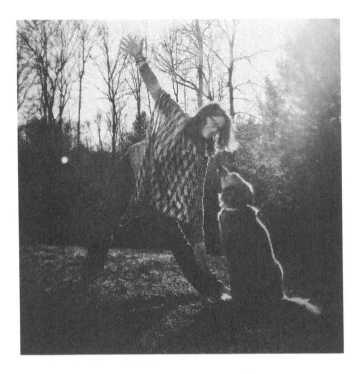

Nancy Alder is a mom, yoga teacher
and writer based in Connecticut. She
teaches yogis to find their wings with
ease through anatomy, acceptance and
humor whether instructing arm balances
or Savasana. She is known for making
the esoteric approachable for all through
intelligent sequencing and language.
Her blog, Flying Yogini, introduced
many readers to the empathetic truths
and funny tales which also narrate her
classes.

Nancy is trained in many styles of yoga ranging from vinyasa to yin and blends all of those influences creatively in her classes which are never the same. Her emphasis on *Sangha*, or community, shows in the way the yogis on her retreats and in her classes become a family. She is 500H trained, and teaches a blend of Buddhism with Forrest, Hatha, and Vinyasa yoga. Her personal practice is about living an eight limbed life; yoga 24/7.

Nancy has been featured in and has written for both *Origin Magazine* and *Mantra Yoga + Health Magazine,* the latter of which she was also an editor. She was a frequent contributor to actress Carrie-Anne Moss's *Annapurna Living*. Her projects have been highlighted by *Yoga Journal* online and her words can be found on noted yoga sites *YogaDork, Gaiam* and *Hugger Mugger*.

When not teaching or writing, Nancy explores the enchanted forest behind her house with her kids whom she calls "the elves," counts the days until the next snowfall and dreams of talking yoga with Jimmy Fallon on The Tonight Show.

Made in the USA
Lexington, KY
15 May 2017